CHAIR YOGA FOR MEN OVER 50

Quick And Simple Workouts For Weight Loss, Strength, Mobility And Balance

Christopher B. Green

TABLE OF CONTENTS

INTRODUCTION 5

CHAPTER 1 7

Understanding Chair Yoga for Men Over 50 7

Benefits of Chair Yoga for Men Over 50 9

Safety Precautions and Guidelines for Chair Yoga 12

CHAPTER 2 15

Proper Attire and Equipment for Chair Yoga 15

BREATHING AND RELAXATION TECHNIQUES 18

Seated Belly Breathing (Diaphragmatic Breathing) 18

Seated Alternate Nostril Breathing (Nadi Shodhana) 19

Seated Forward Fold Breathing 20

Seated Shoulder Roll Breathing 21

Seated Lion's Breath (Simhasana) 22

Seated Equal Breathing (Sama Vritti) 23

Seated Ocean Breath (Ujjayi) 24

Seated Three-Part Breath (Dirga Pranayama) 25

Seated Sighing Breath 26

CHAPTER 3 27

CHAIR YOGA POSES FOR MEN OVER 50 27

Boat Pose Variations 27

Chair Dips 28

Chair Reverse Plank 29

Box Squats 30

Seated Bicycle 31

Leg Circles 32

Leg Extend 33

Knee Taps 34

Leg Stretch 35

Body Twist 36

Arm Reaches 37

Chest Stretch 38

Arm Swings 39

Chair March 40

Knee Extension 41

Seated Tummy Twist 42

Inner Thigh Squeeze 43

Seated Row 44

Standing Leg Raise with Chair 45

Seated Side Bend 46

Forward Fold 47

Front Clap 48

Seated Eagle Pose 49

Leg Raise 50

Warrior II (Seated Variation) 51

Seated Cow Face Pose 53

Seated Mountain Pose 54

Assisted Neck Stretch 55

Seated Hero's Pose 56

The High Altar Side Leans 57

CHAPTER 4 59

28 DAYS CHAIR YOGA FOR MEN OVER 50 59

CHAPTER 5 72

RESOURCES AND EXTRAS 72

Chair Yoga Illustrations 72

Chair Yoga Video 73

Fitness Planner 74

CONCLUSION 85

INTRODUCTION

Mark, a 55-year-old retired engineer, had always been active in his younger years. He used to enjoy long hikes and even played sports on the weekends. But as time went on, Mark found himself struggling with stiff joints, persistent back pain, and a growing sense of frustration as simple movements became more challenging. He missed the freedom and ease of being able to move without discomfort. One day, while chatting with a friend about his struggles, the friend suggested yoga. Mark's first reaction was to laugh it off, he thought yoga was too complicated, especially for someone his age. But then his friend introduced him to chair yoga, a gentle alternative that changed everything for Mark.

Within just a few weeks of practicing chair yoga, Mark felt a remarkable difference. His flexibility improved, his strength increased, and, most importantly, his pain lessened. Mark didn't have to get down on the floor or twist into complicated positions. Instead, using just a sturdy chair, he could perform simple movements that fit his body's needs and capabilities. For the first time in years, Mark felt empowered and confident in his body again.

This guide, ***Chair Yoga for Men Over 50***, is designed for men like Mark who want to regain control of their physical health and feel good in their bodies, but may not feel comfortable with traditional forms of exercise. Chair yoga is a gentle, accessible form of exercise that can help improve your flexibility, strengthen muscles, boost energy levels, and even reduce stress. Whether you are dealing with joint pain, stiffness, or simply want to stay active and improve your mobility, chair yoga offers an easy and effective way to do so right from the comfort of your home.

In this book, you will find step-by-step routines tailored specifically for men over 50. With consistent practice, you'll discover how small, simple movements can make a big difference in how you feel each day. Let's take the first step toward moving better, feeling stronger, and living more comfortably starting with a chair.

CHAPTER 1

Understanding Chair Yoga for Men Over 50

Chair yoga is a modified form of traditional yoga that makes it possible for people with limited mobility, balance issues, or those who are simply uncomfortable with floor-based exercises to enjoy the benefits of yoga. For men over 50, chair yoga can be a game changer. It offers a way to stay active, stretch the muscles, and improve overall well-being without the need to perform complex poses or use yoga mats. Instead, a sturdy chair is the primary tool, making the practice more accessible for men who may be dealing with joint pain, stiffness, or general discomfort from aging.

As we age, it is common for mobility to decrease, leading to more sedentary lifestyles, which can further contribute to muscle weakness, loss of flexibility, and reduced balance. Chair yoga addresses these challenges by focusing on gentle, low-impact movements that gradually increase strength, flexibility, and mobility. The exercises are designed to reduce the strain on your joints while still giving your muscles a workout. This approach helps protect your knees, hips, and back, areas where many men over 50 tend to experience the most discomfort.

One of the primary advantages of chair yoga is that it allows men over 50 to participate in a consistent exercise routine without worrying about the risks of falling or overexerting themselves. Many traditional yoga poses are adapted to the chair, offering stability and support while still engaging the body in beneficial movements. For instance, standing poses can be done with the chair providing support, and seated poses are modified to work the muscles effectively, even while sitting.

Beyond the physical benefits, chair yoga also offers mental and emotional benefits. The practice of mindful breathing, which is central to yoga, helps reduce stress, improve focus, and promote a sense of calm. For men over 50, stress management becomes increasingly important, as life changes such as retirement, family dynamics, or health concerns can cause anxiety. Chair yoga allows you to center your mind and breathe deeply, fostering both physical and emotional balance.

Chair yoga is not just for those who are new to exercise but also for men who want to maintain an active lifestyle despite physical limitations. By focusing on slow, controlled movements and breathing exercises, chair yoga can improve your flexibility, strength, and mental clarity allowing you to age gracefully while staying active and engaged in your daily life.

Benefits of Chair Yoga for Men Over 50

1. Improved Flexibility

Chair yoga helps increase flexibility by gently stretching muscles and joints, which tend to stiffen with age. Men over 50 often face reduced flexibility, leading to discomfort and decreased range of motion. Regular chair yoga sessions can restore and enhance flexibility, making everyday movements easier and reducing the risk of injuries.

2. Enhanced Strength

Chair yoga incorporates poses that engage various muscle groups, building strength without the need for strenuous exercise. This is particularly beneficial for men over 50 who may not be able to perform high-impact workouts. Strengthened muscles support joints, improve posture, and contribute to overall physical stability.

3. Better Balance and Stability

As men age, maintaining balance can become challenging, increasing the risk of falls. Chair yoga focuses on balance through controlled movements and poses. By improving proprioception and core strength, chair yoga enhances overall stability, helping men navigate their daily activities with confidence.

4. Joint Health

Maintaining joint health requires improved circulation and lubrication of the joints, which is what chair yoga's mild motions do. Diseases like arthritis frequently cause men over 50 to have joint pain and stiffness. Chair yoga can alleviate these symptoms by promoting joint flexibility and reducing inflammation.

5. Stress Reduction

Chair yoga incorporates deep breathing and mindfulness, which are effective in reducing stress and anxiety. For men over 50, managing stress is vital for overall health. The meditative aspect of chair yoga helps calm the mind, reduce cortisol levels, and promote a sense of inner peace.

6. Enhanced Mental Clarity

Regular practice of chair yoga can improve mental focus and clarity. The combination of physical movement and mindfulness sharpens cognitive functions, which can decline with age. Men over 50 can benefit from improved memory, concentration, and mental agility, which are essential for both personal and professional life.

7. Cardiovascular Health

While chair yoga is low-impact, it can still provide cardiovascular benefits. The gentle movements increase heart rate moderately, improving cardiovascular health without putting undue stress on the body. This can help men over 50 maintain a healthy heart and reduce the risk of cardiovascular diseases.

8. Digestive Health

Yoga poses in chair yoga can stimulate digestive organs and improve digestion. For men over 50, digestive issues can become more prevalent. Chair yoga promotes better digestion, alleviates constipation, and enhances overall gut health, contributing to improved nutrient absorption and energy levels.

9. Pain Management

Chair yoga is an excellent way to manage chronic pain, which is common in men over 50 due to conditions like arthritis or back pain. The gentle stretching and strengthening exercises reduce muscle tension and improve blood flow, which can alleviate pain and discomfort. Regular practice can lead to long-term pain relief and improved quality of life.

10. Social Interaction

Attending chair yoga sessions might facilitate beneficial social connection. Keeping up with social media is crucial for males over 50's mental and emotional well-being. Chair yoga classes offer a community environment where individuals can connect, share experiences, and support each other, reducing feelings of isolation and promoting a sense of belonging.

Safety Precautions and Guidelines for Chair Yoga

1. Choose the Right Chair

Ensure the chair used for yoga is stable, sturdy, and without wheels. It should have a straight back and provide adequate support. The chair's height should allow your feet to rest flat on the floor, ensuring proper alignment and stability during exercises.

2. Warm-Up Properly

Before starting chair yoga, it's important to warm up the body with gentle movements or stretches. This prepares the muscles and joints, reduces the risk of injury, and improves flexibility. Simple arm circles, neck rolls, and ankle rotations can effectively loosen up the body.

3. Listen to Your Body

Always listen to your body and avoid pushing yourself too hard. If a pose causes pain or significant discomfort, modify it or skip it altogether. Pain is a signal that something is wrong, and ignoring it can lead to injury.

4. Breathe Mindfully

Throughout the session, keep your breathing slow and deep. In addition to improving oxygen flow and relaxation, proper breathing also aids in maintaining a steady beat. Inhale through the nose and exhale through the mouth, coordinating breath with movement for optimal results.

5. Maintain Proper Alignment

Pay attention to body alignment in each pose to prevent strain and injury. Keep the spine straight, shoulders relaxed, and avoid slouching. Proper alignment ensures that the muscles are engaged correctly and reduces unnecessary stress on joints.

6. Use Props and Supports

To improve comfort and stability, use yoga props like cushions, belts, and blocks. Props can facilitate proper alignment and ease the transition into poses, especially for individuals with restricted range of motion or mobility. Don't hesitate to use these aids to modify poses as needed.

7. Stay Hydrated

Keep a bottle of water nearby and stay hydrated, especially during longer sessions. Proper hydration supports muscle function, helps maintain energy levels, and aids in recovery. Drink water before, during, and after the practice to stay refreshed.

8. Avoid Overstretching

While stretching is beneficial, it's crucial to avoid overstretching, which can lead to muscle strains or injuries. Stretch to the point of mild tension but not pain. Gradually increase flexibility over time without forcing the body into uncomfortable positions.

9. Consult with a Healthcare Professional

Before starting a chair yoga program, consult with a healthcare professional, especially if you have pre-existing medical conditions or concerns. A doctor can provide personalized advice and ensure that chair yoga is safe and appropriate for your health needs.

10. Practice Regularly but Rest When Needed

Consistency is key to reaping the benefits of chair yoga, but it's also important to rest when needed. Incorporate regular practice into your routine, but listen to your body and take breaks if you feel fatigued or sore. Balance activity with adequate rest to prevent burnout and overuse injuries.

CHAPTER 2

Proper Attire and Equipment for Chair Yoga

Attire

1. Comfortable Clothing

- Wear loose-fitting, breathable clothes that allow for a full range of motion. Avoid tight or restrictive garments that could hinder movement. Ideal options include athletic shorts, sweatpants, and T-shirts made from moisture-wicking materials to keep you dry and comfortable during the session.

2. Non-Slip Socks or Bare Feet

- Practicing chair yoga barefoot or with non-slip socks provides better grip and stability, reducing the risk of slipping. Non-slip socks are particularly useful if you prefer not to be barefoot, offering both comfort and safety.

3. Supportive Footwear (Optional)

- If you prefer wearing shoes, choose lightweight, flexible footwear with good grip and support. Avoid heavy or rigid shoes that can restrict movement or add unnecessary weight.

4. Layered Clothing

- Consider wearing layers that can be easily added or removed as needed. This allows you to adjust to different temperatures and maintain comfort throughout the session. A light jacket or hoodie can be useful during warm-ups and cool-downs.

Equipment

1. Sturdy Chair

- To enable a greater range of motion, use a solid, non-slip chair without wheels that preferably has a straight back and no arms. Ensure the chair is the right height so that your feet can rest flat on the floor, providing a secure base for exercises.

2. Yoga Mat (Optional)

- Placing a yoga mat under the chair can prevent it from slipping and provide additional cushioning for your feet. This is especially useful on hard surfaces.

3. Yoga Blocks

- Yoga blocks can be used to modify poses and provide additional support. They help maintain proper alignment and can be placed under hands or feet to make stretches more accessible.

4. Yoga Strap

- A yoga strap assists in deepening stretches and improving flexibility. It's particularly beneficial for individuals with limited range of motion, allowing them to achieve proper form without strain.

5. Cushions or Pillows

- Cushions or pillows can be used for added comfort and support. They can be placed on the chair seat to provide additional height or behind the lower back for lumbar support, enhancing posture and alignment.

6. Water Bottle

- Staying hydrated is important during any physical activity. Keep a water bottle nearby to ensure you can drink water before, during, and after your chair yoga session.

7. Towel

- Have a towel handy to wipe away sweat and maintain comfort. A small hand towel can also be used as an additional prop to assist with stretches if a yoga strap is not available.

8. Music or Relaxation App (Optional)

- Playing soothing music or using a relaxation app can enhance the yoga experience by creating a calming environment. This can help with mindfulness and stress reduction during your practice.

BREATHING AND RELAXATION TECHNIQUES

Seated Belly Breathing (Diaphragmatic Breathing)

- **Starting Position:** Place your feet firmly on the ground and sit comfortably in a chair with your back straight. Put one hand on your abdomen and the other on your chest.

- **Steps:**

1. Inhale deeply through your nose, allowing your abdomen to expand while keeping your chest relatively still.

2. Feel your hand on your abdomen rise as you breathe in.

3. Exhale slowly through your mouth, letting your abdomen fall.

4. Repeat the process for 5-10 minutes, focusing on the rise and fall of your abdomen.

- **Repetition:** Practice daily for 5-10 minutes.

- **Purpose:** This method uses the diaphragm more effectively, which helps to expand lung capacity, lower stress levels, and encourage relaxation.

Seated Alternate Nostril Breathing

(Nadi Shodhana)

- Starting Position:

Take a comfortable seat with your shoulders relaxed and your back straight.

- Steps:

1. Close your right nostril with your thumb.

2. Take a deep breath through your left nose.

3. Using your right ring finger, shut your left nostril and open your right.

4. Exhale slowly through your right nostril.

5. Breathe in using your right nostril.

6. Breathe out via your left nostril while closing your right.

7. This completes one cycle.

- Repetition: Perform 5-10 cycles, once or twice daily.

- Purpose: This technique balances the nervous system, reduces stress, and enhances mental clarity.

Seated Forward Fold Breathing

- Starting Position:

Position yourself on a chair's edge, keeping your feet hip-width apart and flat on the ground.

- Steps:

1. Inhale deeply, lengthening your spine.

2. Exhale and slowly hinge forward at the hips, allowing your upper body to drape over your thighs.

3. Let your hands rest on the floor or dangle by your sides.

4. Take several deep breaths in this position, feeling the stretch in your back and legs.

5. Inhale as you slowly rise back to a seated position.

- Repetition: Repeat 3-5 times.

- Purpose: This technique stretches the back and hamstrings, relieves tension, and promotes deep breathing and relaxation.

Seated Shoulder Roll Breathing

- Starting Position:

Sit comfortably with your back straight and feet flat on the floor.

- Steps:

1. Inhale deeply and lift your shoulders up towards your ears.

2. Exhale slowly, rolling your shoulders back and down.

3. Continue this movement, syncing the shoulder rolls with your breath.

4. After several rolls in one direction, switch to rolling your shoulders forward with each inhale and exhale.

- Repetition: Perform 10-15 rolls in each direction.

- Purpose: This technique releases tension in the shoulders and neck, improves posture, and encourages mindful breathing.

Seated Lion's Breath (Simhasana)

- **Starting Position:**

Sit comfortably on a chair with your back straight and feet flat on the floor. Place your hands on your knees with fingers spread wide.

- **Steps:**

1. Inhale deeply through your nose.

2. As you exhale, open your mouth wide and stick out your tongue, extending it down towards your chin.

3. Make a "ha" sound from deep within your abdomen as you exhale forcefully.

4. Relax your face and close your mouth after each exhale.

5. Repeat for 5-7 breaths.

- **Repetition:** Practice once or twice daily for 5-7 breaths.

- **Purpose:** This technique relieves tension in the face and neck, promotes relaxation, and helps release stress and pent-up emotions.

Seated Equal Breathing (Sama Vritti)

- **Starting Position:**

 Sit comfortably with your back straight and feet flat on the floor.

- **Steps:**

   1. Inhale slowly through your nose for a count of four.

   2. Exhale slowly through your nose for a count of four, making the inhale and exhale equal in duration.

   3. Focus on maintaining a steady, even breath.

   4. Gradually increase the count to six or eight if comfortable.

- **Repetition:** Practice for 5-10 minutes daily.

- **Purpose:** This technique helps balance the breath, reduces stress, and promotes a sense of calm and focus.

Seated Ocean Breath (Ujjayi)

- Starting Position:

Sit comfortably on a chair with your back straight and feet flat on the floor.

- Steps:

1. Breathe in deeply through your nostrils while slightly tightening your throat to produce a whispery, gentle sound.

2. Exhale through your nose, maintaining the same constriction in your throat to produce the ocean-like sound.

3. Continue this breath, focusing on the sound and sensation.

- Repetition: Practice for 5-10 minutes.

- Purpose: This technique increases oxygen consumption, promotes relaxation, and helps improve focus and concentration

Seated Three-Part Breath (Dirga Pranayama)

- Starting Position:

Sit comfortably with your back straight and feet flat on the floor.

- Steps:

1. Inhale deeply into your lower abdomen, allowing it to expand fully.

2. Continue to inhale, filling your mid-chest area.

3. Finally, fill your upper chest and collarbone area with air.

4. Exhale slowly in reverse order, emptying the upper chest, mid-chest, and then the lower abdomen.

5. Continue this pattern for several breaths.

- Repetition: Practice for 5-10 minutes daily.

- Purpose: This technique promotes complete and deep breathing, enhances lung capacity, and reduces stress and anxiety.

Seated Sighing Breath

- Starting Position:

Sit comfortably with your back straight and feet flat on the floor.

- Steps:

1. Inhale deeply through your nose.

2. Exhale with an audible sigh through your mouth, releasing tension from your body.

3. Allow your shoulders to drop and relax with each exhale.

4. Repeat for 5-10 breaths.

- Repetition: Practice as needed, particularly when feeling stressed or tense.

- Purpose: This method facilitates relaxation, eases tension, and brings on a sudden feeling of peace and relief.

CHAPTER 3

CHAIR YOGA POSES FOR MEN

OVER 50

Boat Pose Variations

Starting Position:

- Sit on the edge of a sturdy chair with your feet flat on the floor and knees bent at 90 degrees.

- Place your hands on the sides of the chair for support.

Steps:

- Engage your core muscles and lean back slightly while lifting your feet off the floor. Your legs should form a 45-degree angle with the floor.

- Hold this position, balancing on your sit bones while keeping your spine straight.

- For a variation, extend your arms forward at shoulder height, parallel to the floor.

- To intensify the pose, straighten your legs so that your body forms a V shape.

- Hold the pose for 15-30 seconds, then slowly lower your feet back to the floor.

Repetitions:

- Repeat this exercise 3-5 times, holding each pose for 15-30 seconds.

Purpose:

- The Boat Pose strengthens the core muscles, improves balance and stability, and enhances overall body awareness. It's particularly beneficial for men over 50 to build core strength, which supports posture and reduces the risk of back pain.

Chair Dips

Starting Position:

- Sit on the edge of a sturdy chair with your hands gripping the front edge of the seat, fingers pointing forward.

- Extend your legs straight out in front of you with your heels on the floor, keeping a slight bend in your knees.

Steps:

- Slide your hips off the chair while keeping your hands firmly on the seat.

- Lower your body by bending your elbows, keeping them close to your body, until your upper arms are nearly parallel to the floor.

- Push through your palms to lift your body back up to the starting position.

- Keep your shoulders down and back throughout the movement.

Repetitions:

- Perform 10-15 repetitions per set, and aim for 2-3 sets.

Purpose:

- Chair Dips target the triceps, shoulders, and chest muscles. They are effective for building upper body strength, which is crucial for maintaining functional fitness and performing daily activities with ease as men age.

Chair Reverse Plank

Starting Position:

- Sit on the edge of a sturdy chair with your legs extended in front of you and your heels on the floor.

- Place your hands on the edge of the chair, fingers pointing forward.

Steps:

- Engage your core and press through your hands to lift your hips off the chair, forming a straight line from your head to your heels.

- Keep your chest open and shoulders away from your ears.

- Hold this position for 15-30 seconds, focusing on keeping your body in a straight line.

Repetitions:

- Repeat this exercise 3-5 times, holding the plank for 15-30 seconds each time.

Purpose:

- The Chair Reverse Plank strengthens the core, glutes, lower back, and shoulders. This exercise helps improve posture, stability, and overall body strength, which are important for preventing injuries and maintaining mobility as men age.

Box Squats

Starting Position:

- Stand in front of a chair with your feet hip-width apart, toes pointing slightly outward.

- Cross your arms in front of your chest or extend them forward for balance

Steps:

- Push your hips back and bend your knees to lower your body as if you are sitting down in the chair.

- Lightly tap the chair with your glutes without fully sitting down.

- Engage your core and push through your heels to return to the standing position.

- Keep your chest lifted and your back straight throughout the movement.

Repetitions:

- Perform 10-15 repetitions per set, and aim for 2-3 sets.

Purpose:

- Box Squats strengthen the quadriceps, hamstrings, and glutes, which are essential for maintaining lower body strength and mobility. This exercise also helps improve balance and stability, reducing the risk of falls in men over 50.

Seated Bicycle

Starting Position:

- Sit on the edge of a sturdy chair with your feet flat on the floor and knees bent at 90 degrees.

- Place your hands behind your head with elbows pointing outward.

Steps:

- Engage your core and lift your right knee toward your chest while simultaneously twisting your torso to bring your left elbow toward your right knee.

- Return to the starting position and repeat the movement on the opposite side, bringing your right elbow toward your left knee.

- Continue alternating sides in a smooth, controlled motion, as if pedaling a bicycle.

Repetitions:

- Perform 10-15 repetitions per side, and aim for 2-3 sets.

Purpose:

- The Seated Bicycle targets the core muscles, particularly the obliques, while also engaging the hip flexors. This exercise helps improve core strength and rotational stability, which are important for maintaining balance and preventing injuries in daily activities.

Leg Circles

Starting Position:

- Sit comfortably on a sturdy chair with your feet flat on the floor and back straight.

- Place your hands on the sides of the chair for support.

Steps:

- Extend your right leg straight out in front of you, keeping it parallel to the floor.

- Begin making small circles with your leg in a clockwise direction, keeping the movement controlled and smooth.

- After completing a set of circles, switch to counterclockwise circles.

- Lower your leg back to the starting position and repeat with the left leg.

Repetitions:

- Perform 10 circles in each direction per leg, and aim for 2-3 sets.

Purpose:

- Leg Circles improve hip mobility, strengthen the quadriceps, and enhance coordination. This exercise helps maintain flexibility and range of motion in the hips, which is vital for activities like walking and climbing stairs as men age.

Leg Extend

Starting Position:

- Sit on a sturdy chair with your feet flat on the floor and back straight.

- Place your hands on the sides of the chair for support.

Steps:

- Extend your right leg straight out in front of you, keeping your foot flexed and your leg parallel to the floor.

- Hold the extended position for a few seconds, feeling the contraction in your quadriceps.

- Slowly lower your leg back to the starting position.

- Repeat with the left leg.

Repetitions:

- Perform 10-15 repetitions per leg, and aim for 2-3 sets.

Purpose:

- Leg Extend strengthens the quadriceps, which are important for knee stability and overall leg strength. This exercise is beneficial for maintaining functional mobility and reducing the risk of knee injuries in men over 50.

Knee Taps

Starting Position:

- Sit on a sturdy chair with your feet flat on the floor and back straight.

- Place your hands on the sides of the chair for support.

Steps:

- Lift your right knee toward your chest while keeping your back straight.

- As you lift your knee, tap it gently with your left hand.

- Lower your right leg back to the starting position and repeat with your left knee and right hand.

- Continue alternating sides in a controlled motion.

Repetitions:

- Perform 10-15 repetitions per side, and aim for 2-3 sets.

Purpose:

- Knee Taps engage the core, hip flexors, and lower abdominal muscles. This exercise improves coordination, balance, and lower body strength, all of which are essential for maintaining mobility and stability in older adults.

Leg Stretch

Starting Position:

- Sit on the edge of a sturdy chair with your feet flat on the floor and knees bent at 90 degrees.

- Keep your back straight and hands resting on your thighs.

Steps:

- Extend your right leg straight out in front of you, keeping your foot flexed.

- Slowly lean forward from your hips, reaching toward your extended foot while keeping your back straight.

- Hold the stretch for 15-30 seconds, feeling the stretch in your hamstrings.

- Return to the starting position and repeat with the left leg.

Repetitions:

- Perform 2-3 stretches per leg, holding each stretch for 15-30 seconds.

Purpose:

- Leg Stretch improves hamstring flexibility, enhances circulation, and helps prevent muscle tightness. Regular stretching is crucial for maintaining flexibility and reducing the risk of muscle strains and injuries in men over 50.

Body Twist

Starting Position:

- Sit on a sturdy chair with your feet flat on the floor and back straight.

- Place your hands on your thighs or the sides of the chair for support.

Steps:

- Engage your core and gently twist your torso to the right, reaching your left hand across to the outside of your right thigh.

- Hold the twist for a few seconds, feeling the stretch along your spine and in your oblique muscles.

- Slowly return to the center and repeat the twist to the left, reaching your right hand across to the outside of your left thigh.

Repetitions:

- Perform 5-10 twists per side, and aim for 2-3 sets.

Purpose:

- Body Twist improves spinal mobility, enhances flexibility in the obliques, and helps release tension in the lower back. This exercise is beneficial for maintaining a healthy spine and reducing stiffness, which is important for overall mobility and comfort in daily activities.

Arm Reaches

Starting Position:

- Sit on a sturdy chair with your feet flat on the floor and back straight.

- Relax your shoulders and place your hands on your thighs.

Steps:

- Extend your right arm straight up toward the ceiling, reaching as high as you can without lifting your shoulder.

- Hold the reach for a few seconds, feeling the stretch along your side and through your arm.

- Lower your right arm and repeat the movement with your left arm.

- For a variation, you can reach both arms overhead simultaneously and then alternate reaching up and to the side.

Repetitions:

- Perform 10-15 reaches per arm, and aim for 2-3 sets.

Purpose:

- Arm Reaches stretch the muscles along the sides of your torso, shoulders, and upper back. This exercise helps improve flexibility, increase range of motion in the shoulders, and alleviate stiffness, which is particularly beneficial for men over 50 to maintain upper body mobility.

Chest Stretch

Starting Position:

- Sit on a sturdy chair with your feet flat on the floor and back straight.

- Place your hands on your thighs.

Steps:

- Clasp your hands behind your back and gently squeeze your shoulder blades together, lifting your chest and extending your arms backward.

- Keep your shoulders down and away from your ears as you open up your chest.

- Hold the stretch for 15-30 seconds, breathing deeply.

Repetitions:

- Perform 2-3 chest stretches, holding each stretch for 15-30 seconds.

Purpose:

- The Chest Stretch helps open up the chest, counteracting the effects of slouching or rounded shoulders. It improves posture, increases flexibility in the chest and shoulders, and can alleviate upper back and neck tension.

Arm Swings

Starting Position:

- Sit or stand (depending on your comfort) with your feet shoulder-width apart and arms relaxed at your sides.

- Keep your back straight and core engaged.

Steps:

- Swing your arms forward and up to shoulder height, then back and down in a smooth, controlled motion.

- Continue swinging your arms, focusing on a full range of motion through the shoulders.

- For an added challenge, alternate arm swings by bringing one arm forward while the other swings back.

Repetitions:

- Perform 15-20 arm swings, and aim for 2-3 sets.

Purpose:

- Arm Swings help warm up the shoulder joints, increase circulation, and enhance flexibility in the upper body. This exercise is great for improving coordination and maintaining shoulder mobility, which is crucial for performing daily tasks comfortably.

Chair March

Starting Position:

- Sit on a sturdy chair with your feet flat on the floor and back straight.

- Place your hands on the sides of the chair for support.

Steps:

- Lift your right knee toward your chest as if you are marching in place.

- Lower your right leg back to the floor and immediately lift your left knee toward your chest.

- Continue alternating legs in a controlled, rhythmic motion, as if marching while seated.

- Maintain a steady pace and keep your core engaged throughout the exercise.

Repetitions:

- Perform 20-30 marches, and aim for 2-3 sets.

Purpose:

- Chair Marches improve cardiovascular endurance, enhance coordination, and strengthen the hip flexors and lower abdominal muscles. This low-impact exercise is excellent for maintaining overall fitness and promoting circulation, especially in men over 50.

Knee Extension

Starting Position:

- Sit on a sturdy chair with your feet flat on the floor and back straight.

- Place your hands on the sides of the chair for support.

Steps:

- Extend your right leg straight out in front of you, keeping your foot flexed and your leg parallel to the floor.

- Hold the extended position for a few seconds, feeling the contraction in your quadriceps.

- Slowly lower your leg back to the starting position.

- Repeat with the left leg.

Repetitions:

- Perform 10-15 repetitions per leg, and aim for 2-3 sets.

Purpose:

- Knee Extensions strengthen the quadriceps and improve knee stability. This exercise is crucial for maintaining leg strength and joint health, helping to reduce the risk of knee injuries and support functional movement in men over 50.

Seated Tummy Twist

Starting Position:

- Sit on a sturdy chair with your feet flat on the floor and back straight.

- Place your hands on your thighs or hold a small, light object (like a ball) in front of your chest.

Steps:

- Engage your core and gently twist your torso to the right, keeping your hips and legs stable.

- As you twist, move your hands or the object across your body toward the outside of your right thigh.

- Hold the twist for a moment, then slowly return to the center.

- Repeat the twist to the left side.

Repetitions:

- Perform 10-15 twists per side, and aim for 2-3 sets.

Purpose:

- The Seated Tummy Twist targets the oblique muscles and improves rotational stability in the core. This exercise helps enhance flexibility, strengthen the core, and improve spinal mobility, which is vital for maintaining balance and preventing injuries in men over 50.

Inner Thigh Squeeze

Starting Position:

- Sit on a sturdy chair with your feet flat on the floor and back straight.

- Place a small, firm cushion or yoga block between your knees.

Steps:

- Squeeze the cushion or block between your knees by engaging your inner thigh muscles.

- Hold the squeeze for 5-10 seconds, focusing on keeping the rest of your body relaxed.

- Release the squeeze slowly and repeat.

Repetitions:

- Perform 10-15 squeezes, and aim for 2-3 sets.

Purpose:

- The Inner Thigh Squeeze strengthens the adductor muscles (inner thighs), which are important for stabilizing the hips and knees. This exercise helps maintain lower body strength and balance, which is essential for daily activities and reducing the risk of falls in men over 50.

Seated Row

Starting Position:

- Sit on a sturdy chair with your feet flat on the floor and back straight.

- Hold a resistance band or light weights with your arms extended in front of you at shoulder height.

Steps:

- Engage your back muscles and pull the resistance band or weights toward your torso, bending your elbows and squeezing your shoulder blades together.

- Keep your elbows close to your body as you pull, and avoid shrugging your shoulders.

- Slowly return to the starting position, controlling the movement.

Repetitions:

- Perform 10-15 repetitions, and aim for 2-3 sets.

Purpose:

- The Seated Row strengthens the upper back, shoulders, and arms. This exercise helps improve posture, enhances upper body strength, and supports the muscles needed for lifting and pulling movements, which are important for functional fitness in men over 50.

Standing Leg Raise with Chair

Starting Position:

- Stand behind a sturdy chair, placing your hands on the chair for support.

- Position your feet hip-width apart and keep your back straight.

Steps:

- Engage your core and slowly lift your right leg straight out behind you while keeping your leg straight and your foot flexed.

- As you lift your leg, avoid arching your back or leaning forward; focus on using your gluteal muscles to raise your leg.

- Hold the raised leg position for a few seconds, keeping your hips level.

- Slowly lower your right leg back to the starting position.

- Repeat the movement with your left leg.

Repetitions:

- Perform 10-15 leg lifts per leg, and aim for 2-3 sets.

Purpose:

- This exercise strengthens the glutes, hamstrings, and lower back muscles. It also improves balance and stability in the lower body, which is essential for maintaining functional strength and preventing falls as men age. The support of the chair helps focus on proper form, making this exercise accessible and safe for men over 50.

Seated Side Bend

Starting Position:

- Sit on a sturdy chair with your feet flat on the floor and back straight.

- Place your hands at the back of your head, elbows pointing outward.

Steps:

- Engage your core and gently bend to the right, bringing your right elbow toward your hip while keeping your left elbow pointing upward.

- Hold the side bend for a moment, feeling the stretch along your left side.

- Slowly return to the center and repeat the movement on the left side.

- Focus on using your oblique muscles to control the movement.

Repetitions:

- Perform 10-15 bends per side, and aim for 2-3 sets.

Purpose:

- The Side Bend with Hands at the Back of Your Head stretches the obliques and strengthens the lateral muscles of the torso. This exercise helps improve flexibility, enhances core strength, and supports proper spinal alignment, which are important for maintaining a healthy back and reducing the risk of injury.

Forward Fold

Starting Position:

- Sit on the edge of a sturdy chair with your feet flat on the floor and knees hip-width apart.

- Keep your back straight and hands resting on your thighs.

Steps:

- Inhale deeply, then as you exhale, gently hinge forward from your hips, reaching your hands toward your feet or the floor.

- Allow your head and neck to relax, letting your upper body hang naturally.

- Hold this position for 15-30 seconds, breathing deeply.

- Slowly roll up to the starting position, stacking your spine one vertebra at a time.

Repetitions:

- Perform 2-3 forward folds, holding each fold for 15-30 seconds.

Purpose:

- The Forward Fold stretches the hamstrings, lower back, and spine, helping to release tension and improve flexibility. This exercise is particularly beneficial for relieving tightness in the back and promoting relaxation, which is essential for men over 50 to maintain a flexible and pain-free spine.

Front Clap

Starting Position:

- Sit or stand with your feet shoulder-width apart, back straight, and arms relaxed at your sides.

Steps:

- Extend your arms straight out in front of you at shoulder height, palms facing each other.

- Clap your hands together in front of you, then quickly return them to the starting position.

- Continue clapping your hands in a controlled, rhythmic motion.

Repetitions:

- Perform 15-20 claps, and aim for 2-3 sets.

Purpose:

- Front Claps engage the chest, shoulders, and arms, helping to improve upper body coordination and strength. This exercise also increases circulation and warms up the upper body muscles, making it a good preparatory movement for more intense exercises.

Seated Eagle Pose

Starting Position:

- Sit on a sturdy chair with your feet flat on the floor and back straight.

- Extend your arms in front of you at shoulder height, palms facing each other.

Steps:

- Cross your right arm over your left at the elbows, and then bend your elbows so your forearms are vertical, and your hands face each other.

- If possible, wrap your forearms around each other so your palms touch. If this is difficult, simply press the backs of your hands together.

- Lift your elbows slightly while keeping your shoulders down, feeling the stretch in your upper back and shoulders.

- Hold the position for 15-30 seconds, then gently release and switch sides by crossing your left arm over your right.

Repetitions:

- Hold the Seated Eagle Pose for 15-30 seconds on each side, and aim for 2-3 sets.

Purpose:

- The Seated Eagle Pose stretches the shoulders, upper back, and neck, helping to relieve tension and improve flexibility in these areas. This pose also enhances focus and concentration, making it a calming exercise for men over 50.

Leg Raise

Starting Position:

- Sit on a sturdy chair with your feet flat on the floor and back straight.

- Place your hands on the sides of the chair for support.

Steps:

- Engage your core and extend your right leg straight out in front of you, keeping your foot flexed.

- Slowly lift your leg a few inches off the floor, holding the position for a few seconds.

- Lower your leg back to the starting position in a controlled manner.

- Repeat with the left leg.

Repetitions:

- Perform 10-15 leg raises per leg, and aim for 2-3 sets.

Purpose:

- Leg Raises strengthen the quadriceps and hip flexors, which are important for maintaining lower body strength and stability. This exercise also helps improve balance and coordination, which are crucial for preventing falls and maintaining mobility as men age.

Warrior II (Seated Variation)

Starting Position:

- Sit on the edge of a sturdy chair with your feet flat on the floor, knees bent at 90 degrees, and back straight.

- Position your feet wider than hip-width apart, aligning your knees with your ankles.

- Extend your arms out to the sides at shoulder height, palms facing down.

Steps:

- Turn your right foot out to the side, aligning it with your right knee, while keeping your left foot firmly planted on the floor.

- Engage your core and gently twist your torso to the right, keeping your arms extended and parallel to the floor.

- Focus on lengthening your spine and maintaining an open chest as you hold the position.

- Hold the pose for 15-30 seconds, breathing deeply.

- Return to the starting position and repeat on the opposite side by turning your left foot out and twisting to the left.

Repetitions:

- Hold the Warrior II pose for 15-30 seconds on each side, and aim for 2-3 sets.

Purpose:

- The Seated Warrior II variation strengthens the legs, arms, and core muscles while improving balance and stability. This pose also opens the hips and stretches the inner thighs, enhancing flexibility and joint health. It's particularly beneficial for men over 50 to maintain lower body strength, improve posture, and support overall mobility.

Seated Cow Face Pose

Starting Position:

- Sit on a sturdy chair with your feet flat on the floor and back straight.

- Place your hands on your thighs.

Steps:

- Cross your right leg over your left, bringing your right knee directly on top of your left knee.

- Inhale and raise your right arm above your head.

- Bend your right elbow and reach your right hand down your back.

- Simultaneously, bring your left arm behind your back and try to clasp your right hand or reach as close as possible. If this is challenging, use a strap or towel to bridge the gap between your hands.

- Hold the position for 15-30 seconds, breathing deeply.

- Gently release and switch sides by crossing your left leg over your right and switching arm positions.

Repetitions:

- Hold the Seated Cow Face Pose for 15-30 seconds on each side, and aim for 2-3 sets.

Purpose:

- The Seated Cow Face Pose stretches the shoulders, triceps, hips, and thighs, helping to increase flexibility and release tension in these areas. It's particularly beneficial for improving shoulder mobility and relieving tightness in the hips and legs.

Seated Mountain Pose

Starting Position:

- Sit tall on a sturdy chair with your feet flat on the floor, knees bent at 90 degrees, and back straight.

- Rest your hands on your thighs with palms facing down.

Steps:

- Inhale deeply and lengthen your spine, imagining a line of energy extending from the top of your head to your tailbone.

- Press your feet firmly into the floor and engage your core muscles.

- Extend your arms overhead with palms facing each other, keeping your shoulders relaxed and away from your ears.

- Hold the pose for several breaths, focusing on maintaining alignment and balance.

Repetitions:

- Hold the Seated Mountain Pose for 5-10 breaths, and repeat 2-3 times.

Purpose:

- The Seated Mountain Pose helps improve posture, strengthen the core, and promote a sense of grounding and stability. It's a foundational pose that encourages alignment and body awareness, making it a great starting point for any seated yoga practice.

Assisted Neck Stretch

Starting Position:

- Sit on a sturdy chair with your feet flat on the floor and back straight.

- Relax your arms at your sides.

Steps:

- Gently place your right hand on the left side of your head, just above your ear.

- Slowly tilt your head to the right, guiding it with your hand until you feel a gentle stretch along the left side of your neck.

- Hold the stretch for 15-30 seconds, breathing deeply.

- Return to the center and repeat on the opposite side by placing your left hand on the right side of your head and tilting your head to the left.

Repetitions:

- Hold the Assisted Neck Stretch for 15-30 seconds on each side, and aim for 2-3 sets.

Purpose:

- The Assisted Neck Stretch helps relieve tension in the neck and shoulders, improving flexibility and reducing stiffness. This stretch is particularly useful for alleviating discomfort from prolonged sitting or stress.

Seated Hero's Pose

Starting Position:

- Sit on a sturdy chair with your feet flat on the floor and back straight.

- Position your knees slightly wider than hip-width apart.

Steps:

- Slide to the edge of the chair and let your hips sink slightly between your legs, allowing your thighs to rest on the chair.

- Keep your back straight and core engaged as you bring your hands to your knees or thighs.

- Hold the position for several breaths, focusing on lengthening your spine and opening your hips.

Repetitions:

- Hold the Seated Hero's Pose for 15-30 seconds, and repeat 2-3 times.

Purpose:

- The Seated Hero's Pose stretches the quadriceps and hip flexors while promoting better posture and spinal alignment. It's beneficial for men over 50 to maintain hip flexibility and reduce tension in the lower back and legs.

The High Altar Side Leans

Starting Position:

- Sit on a sturdy chair with your feet flat on the floor and back straight.

- Clasp your hands together in front of your chest, then extend your arms overhead, palms facing up.

Steps:

- Inhale deeply and lengthen your spine, reaching your arms upward as high as possible.

- As you exhale, gently lean to the right, feeling a stretch along the left side of your torso.

- Hold the side lean for a few breaths, then return to the center.

- Repeat the movement by leaning to the left, stretching the right side of your torso.

Repetitions:

- Perform 5-10 side leans per side, holding each lean for 3-5 breaths.

Purpose:

- The High Altar Side Leans stretch the sides of the torso, including the obliques and intercostal muscles. This exercise helps improve flexibility in the spine and ribcage, enhances lateral movement, and can relieve tension in the lower back and sides, making it a beneficial addition to any seated yoga routine.

CHAPTER 4

28 DAYS CHAIR YOGA FOR MEN OVER 50

Day 1:

1. Seated Belly Breathing (Diaphragmatic Breathing) (page18)

2. Seated Shoulder Roll Breathing (page 21)

3. Seated Mountain Pose (page 54)

4. Seated Tummy Twist (page 42)

5. Arm Reaches (page 37)

6. Seated Forward Fold Breathing (page 20)

Day 2:

1. Knee Extension (page 41)

2. Seated Equal Breathing (Sama Vritti) (page 23)

3. Seated Side Bend (page 46)

4. Leg Circles (page 32)

5. Chest Stretch (page 38)

6. Seated Hero's Pose (page 56)

Day 3:

1. Seated Alternate Nostril Breathing (Nadi Shodhana) (page 19)

2. Seated Ocean Breath (Ujjayi) (page 24)

3. Forward Fold (page 47)

4. Arm Swings (page 39)

5. Chair March (page 40)

6. Assisted Neck Stretch (page 55)

Day 4:

1. Seated Three-Part Breath (Dirga Pranayama) (page 25)

2. Seated Sighing Breath (page 26)

3. Inner Thigh Squeeze (page 43)

4. Leg Extend (page 33)

5. Seated Row (page 44)

6. The High Altar Side Leans (page 57)

Day 5:

1. Seated Lion's Breath (Simhasana) (page 22)

2. Seated Equal Breathing (Sama Vritti) (page 23)

3. Knee Taps (page 34)

4. Seated Bicycle (page 31)

5. Arm Reaches (page 37)

6. Seated Cow Face Pose (page 53)

Day 6:

1. Seated Belly Breathing (Diaphragmatic Breathing) (page 18)

2. Seated Ocean Breath (Ujjayi) (page 24)

3. Leg Stretch (page 35)

4. Chest Stretch (page 38)

5. Chair March (page 40)

6. Warrior II (Seated Variation) (page 51)

Day 7:

1. Knee Extension (page 41)

2. Seated Forward Fold Breathing (page 20)

3. Leg Raise (page 50)

4. Arm Swings (page 39)

5. Seated Mountain Pose (page 54)

6. Assisted Neck Stretch (page 55)

Day 8:

1. Seated Three-Part Breath (Dirga Pranayama) (page 25)

2. Seated Lion's Breath (Simhasana) (page 22)

3. Seated Row (page 44)

4. Chair Dips (page 28)

5. Leg Circles (page 32)

6. Seated Side Bend (page 46)

7. Boat Pose Variation (page 27)

Day 9:

1. Seated Alternate Nostril Breathing (Nadi Shodhana) (page 19)

2. Seated Equal Breathing (Sama Vritti) (page 23)

3. Leg Extend (page 33)

4. Chair Reverse Plank (page 29)

5. Arm Reaches (page 37)

6. Forward Fold (page 47)

Day 10:

1. Seated Belly Breathing (Diaphragmatic Breathing) (page 18)

2. Seated Ocean Breath (Ujjayi) (page 24)

3. Knee Taps (page 34)

4. Box Squats (page 30)

5. Seated Hero's Pose (page 56)

6. The High Altar Side Leans (page 57)

Day 11:

1. Front Clap (page 48)

2. Seated Forward Fold Breathing (page 20)

3. Inner Thigh Squeeze (page 43)

4. Leg Stretch (page 35)

5. Seated Eagle Pose (page 49)

6. Assisted Neck Stretch (page 55)

Day 12:

1. Seated Three-Part Breath (Dirga Pranayama) (page 25)

2. Seated Sighing Breath (page 26)

3. Seated Row (page 44)

4. Seated Bicycle (page 31)

5. Seated Mountain Pose (page 54)

6. Arm Swings (page 39)

Day 13:

1. Seated Lion's Breath (Simhasana) (page 22)

2. Seated Equal Breathing (Sama Vritti) (page 23)

3. Knee Extension (page 41)

4. Chair Dips (page 28)

5. Seated Side Bend (page 46)

6. Seated Cow Face Pose (page 53)

Day 14:

1. Seated Belly Breathing (Diaphragmatic Breathing) (page 18)

2. Seated Ocean Breath (Ujjayi) (page 24)

3. Leg Raise (page 50)

4. Arm Reaches (page 37)

5. Forward Fold (page 47)

6. Warrior II (Seated Variation) (page 51)

7. Boat Pose Variation (page 27)

Day 15:

1. Seated Tummy Twist (page 42)

2. Seated Forward Fold Breathing (page 20)

3. Leg Extend (page 33)

4. Chair Reverse Plank (page 29)

5. Seated Hero's Pose (page 56)

6. The High Altar Side Leans (page 57)

Day 16:

1. Seated Three-Part Breath (Dirga Pranayama) (page 25)

2. Seated Lion's Breath (Simhasana) (page 22)

3. Seated Row (page 44)

4. Knee Taps (page 34)

5. Seated Eagle Pose (page 49)

6. Assisted Neck Stretch (page 55)

Day 17:

1. Seated Alternate Nostril Breathing (Nadi Shodhana) (page 19)

2. Seated Equal Breathing (Sama Vritti) (page 23)

3. Inner Thigh Squeeze (page 43)

4. Leg Stretch (page 35)

5. Arm Swings (page 39)

6. Seated Mountain Pose (page 54)

Day 18:

1. Seated Belly Breathing (Diaphragmatic Breathing) (page 18)

2. Seated Ocean Breath (Ujjayi) (page 24)

3. Chair March (page 40)

4. Box Squats (page 30)

5. Seated Cow Face Pose (page 53)

6. Forward Fold (page 47)

Day 19:

1. Knee Extension (page 41)

2. Seated Forward Fold Breathing (page 20)

3. Leg Circles (page 32)

4. Chair Dips (page 28)

5. Seated Side Bend (page 46)

6. Seated Hero's Pose (page 56)

Day 20:

1. Seated Three-Part Breath (Dirga Pranayama) (page 25)

2. Seated Sighing Breath (page 26)

3. Seated Row (page 44)

4. Leg Raise (page 50)

5. Arm Reaches (page 37)

6. Assisted Neck Stretch (page 55)

Day 21:

1. Seated Lion's Breath (Simhasana) (page 22)

2. Seated Equal Breathing (Sama Vritti) (page 23)

3. Knee Extension (page 41)

4. Chair March (page 40)

5. Warrior II (Seated Variation) (page 51)

6. The High Altar Side Leans (page 57)

Day 22:

1. Seated Belly Breathing (Diaphragmatic Breathing) (page 18)

2. Seated Ocean Breath (Ujjayi) (page 24)

3. Leg Extend (page 33)

4. Chair Reverse Plank (page 29)

5. Seated Mountain Pose (page 54)

6. Forward Fold (page 47)

Day 23:

1. Knee Extension (page 41)

2. Seated Forward Fold Breathing (page 20)

3. Seated Bicycle (page 31)

4. Leg Stretch (page 35)

5. Arm Swings (page 39)

6. Seated Hero's Pose (page 56)

Day 24:

1. Seated Three-Part Breath (Dirga Pranayama) (page 25)

2. Seated Sighing Breath (page 26)

3. Seated Row (page 44)

4. Leg Circles (page 32)

5. Seated Cow Face Pose (page 53)

6. Assisted Neck Stretch (page 55)

Day 25:

1. Seated Lion's Breath (Simhasana) (page 22)

2. Seated Equal Breathing (Sama Vritti) (page 23)

3. Chair Dips (page 28)

4. Knee Taps (page 34)

5. Arm Reaches (page 37)

6. The High Altar Side Leans (page 57)

Day 26:

1. Seated Belly Breathing (Diaphragmatic Breathing) (page 18)

2. Seated Ocean Breath (Ujjayi) (page 24)

3. Leg Raise (page 50)

4. Seated Row (page 44)

5. Forward Fold (page 47)

6. Warrior II (Seated Variation) (page 51)

Day 27:

1. Standing Leg Raise With Chair (page 45)

2. Seated Forward Fold Breathing (page 20)

3. Knee Extension (page 41)

4. Box Squats (page 30)

5. Seated Side Bend (page 46)

6. Seated Eagle Pose (page 49)

Day 28:

1. Seated Three-Part Breath (Dirga Pranayama) (page 25)

2. Seated Sighing Breath (page 26)

3. Chair March (page 40)

4. Leg Stretch (page 35)

5. Seated Mountain Pose (page 54)

6. Assisted Neck Stretch (page 55)

7. Boat Pose Variation (page 27)

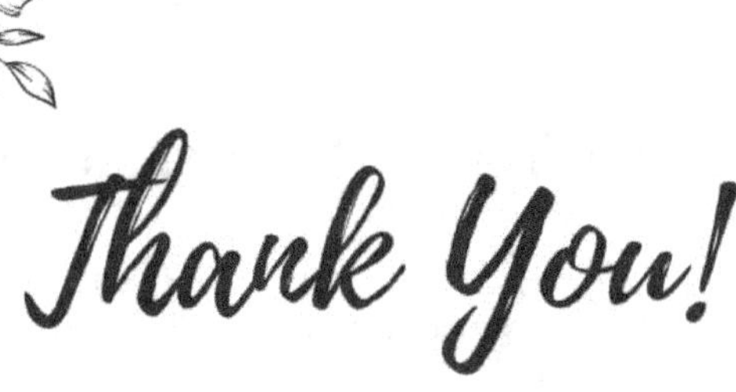

Thank You!

Thank you so much for taking the time to explore this guide. Your feedback is incredibly valuable and helps others discover and benefit from this book. If you found the recipes and tips helpful, I'd truly appreciate it if you could take a moment to leave a review. Your thoughts not only assist others in making their decision but also help me continue creating content that serves you better. Thank you for your support!

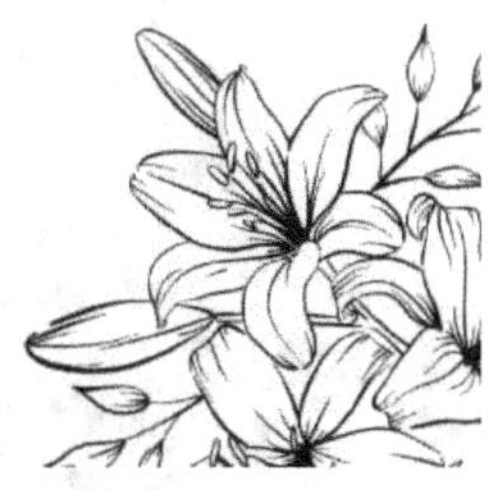

CHAPTER 5

RESOURCES AND EXTRAS

Chair Yoga Illustrations

SCAN THIS CODE TO GET ACCESS TO THE IMAGES OF EACH EXERCISE

How To Scan A QR Code

1. Open your Camera App

2. Point the camera at the QR code.

3. Tap the link or notification that appears and you're done!

Note: If scanning doesn't work, refocus, adjust lighting, or use a dedicated QR scanning app.

Chair Yoga Video

SCAN THIS QR CODE TO GET ACCESS TO THE VIDEO

How To Scan A QR Code

1. Open your Camera App

2. Point the camera at the QR code.

3. Tap the link or notification that appears

Done! You've accessed the QR content

Note: If scanning doesn't work, refocus, adjust lighting, or use a dedicated QR scanning app.

FITNESS PLANNER

DATE:		DURATION:

CHAIR YOGA POSES	SET 1		SET 2		SET 3		SET 4		SET 5	
	WEIGHT	REPS	WEIGHT	REPS	WEIGHT	REPS	WEIGHT	REPS	WEIGHT	REPS

DATE:		DURATION:

CHAIR YOGA POSES	SET 1		SET 2		SET 3		SET 4		SET 5	
	WEIGHT	REPS	WEIGHT	REPS	WEIGHT	REPS	WEIGHT	REPS	WEIGHT	REPS

FITNESS PLANNER

DATE:		DURATION:

CHAIR YOGA POSES	SET 1		SET 2		SET 3		SET 4		SET 5	
	WEIGHT	REPS	WEIGHT	REPS	WEIGHT	REPS	WEIGHT	REPS	WEIGHT	REPS

DATE:		DURATION:

CHAIR YOGA POSES	SET 1		SET 2		SET 3		SET 4		SET 5	
	WEIGHT	REPS	WEIGHT	REPS	WEIGHT	REPS	WEIGHT	REPS	WEIGHT	REPS

FITNESS PLANNER

DATE:		DURATION:

CHAIR YOGA POSES	SET 1		SET 2		SET 3		SET 4		SET 5	
	WEIGHT	REPS	WEIGHT	REPS	WEIGHT	REPS	WEIGHT	REPS	WEIGHT	REPS

DATE:		DURATION:

CHAIR YOGA POSES	SET 1		SET 2		SET 3		SET 4		SET 5	
	WEIGHT	REPS	WEIGHT	REPS	WEIGHT	REPS	WEIGHT	REPS	WEIGHT	REPS

FITNESS PLANNER

DATE:		DURATION:

CHAIR YOGA POSES	SET 1		SET 2		SET 3		SET 4		SET 5	
	WEIGHT	REPS	WEIGHT	REPS	WEIGHT	REPS	WEIGHT	REPS	WEIGHT	REPS

DATE:		DURATION:

CHAIR YOGA POSES	SET 1		SET 2		SET 3		SET 4		SET 5	
	WEIGHT	REPS	WEIGHT	REPS	WEIGHT	REPS	WEIGHT	REPS	WEIGHT	REPS

FITNESS PLANNER

DATE:		DURATION:

CHAIR YOGA POSES	SET 1		SET 2		SET 3		SET 4		SET 5	
	WEIGHT	REPS	WEIGHT	REPS	WEIGHT	REPS	WEIGHT	REPS	WEIGHT	REPS

DATE:		DURATION:

CHAIR YOGA POSES	SET 1		SET 2		SET 3		SET 4		SET 5	
	WEIGHT	REPS	WEIGHT	REPS	WEIGHT	REPS	WEIGHT	REPS	WEIGHT	REPS

FITNESS PLANNER

DATE:		DURATION:

CHAIR YOGA POSES	SET 1		SET 2		SET 3		SET 4		SET 5	
	WEIGHT	REPS	WEIGHT	REPS	WEIGHT	REPS	WEIGHT	REPS	WEIGHT	REPS

DATE:		DURATION:

CHAIR YOGA POSES	SET 1		SET 2		SET 3		SET 4		SET 5	
	WEIGHT	REPS	WEIGHT	REPS	WEIGHT	REPS	WEIGHT	REPS	WEIGHT	REPS

FITNESS PLANNER

DATE:		DURATION:

CHAIR YOGA POSES	SET 1		SET 2		SET 3		SET 4		SET 5	
	WEIGHT	REPS	WEIGHT	REPS	WEIGHT	REPS	WEIGHT	REPS	WEIGHT	REPS

DATE:		DURATION:

CHAIR YOGA POSES	SET 1		SET 2		SET 3		SET 4		SET 5	
	WEIGHT	REPS	WEIGHT	REPS	WEIGHT	REPS	WEIGHT	REPS	WEIGHT	REPS

FITNESS PLANNER

DATE:		DURATION:

CHAIR YOGA POSES	SET 1		SET 2		SET 3		SET 4		SET 5	
	WEIGHT	REPS	WEIGHT	REPS	WEIGHT	REPS	WEIGHT	REPS	WEIGHT	REPS

DATE:		DURATION:

CHAIR YOGA POSES	SET 1		SET 2		SET 3		SET 4		SET 5	
	WEIGHT	REPS	WEIGHT	REPS	WEIGHT	REPS	WEIGHT	REPS	WEIGHT	REPS

FITNESS PLANNER

DATE:		DURATION:

CHAIR YOGA POSES	SET 1		SET 2		SET 3		SET 4		SET 5	
	WEIGHT	REPS	WEIGHT	REPS	WEIGHT	REPS	WEIGHT	REPS	WEIGHT	REPS

DATE:		DURATION:

CHAIR YOGA POSES	SET 1		SET 2		SET 3		SET 4		SET 5	
	WEIGHT	REPS	WEIGHT	REPS	WEIGHT	REPS	WEIGHT	REPS	WEIGHT	REPS

FITNESS PLANNER

DATE:		DURATION:

CHAIR YOGA POSES	SET 1		SET 2		SET 3		SET 4		SET 5	
	WEIGHT	REPS	WEIGHT	REPS	WEIGHT	REPS	WEIGHT	REPS	WEIGHT	REPS

DATE:		DURATION:

CHAIR YOGA POSES	SET 1		SET 2		SET 3		SET 4		SET 5	
	WEIGHT	REPS	WEIGHT	REPS	WEIGHT	REPS	WEIGHT	REPS	WEIGHT	REPS

FITNESS PLANNER

DATE:		DURATION:

CHAIR YOGA POSES	SET 1		SET 2		SET 3		SET 4		SET 5	
	WEIGHT	REPS	WEIGHT	REPS	WEIGHT	REPS	WEIGHT	REPS	WEIGHT	REPS

DATE:		DURATION:

CHAIR YOGA POSES	SET 1		SET 2		SET 3		SET 4		SET 5	
	WEIGHT	REPS	WEIGHT	REPS	WEIGHT	REPS	WEIGHT	REPS	WEIGHT	REPS

CONCLUSION

As men age, maintaining physical fitness, mental sharpness, and emotional balance becomes increasingly important. Chair yoga presents an accessible and effective solution, offering a myriad of benefits tailored to the needs of men over 50. This mild practice is perfect for anyone who have mobility limitations, joint pain, or just want a low-impact workout because it adapts basic yoga poses to a seated position. You can improve your flexibility, strength, balance, and general well-being by including chair yoga into your daily practice. This will help you age gracefully and vibrantly.

Chair yoga targets key areas often affected by aging, such as the joints, muscles, and cardiovascular system. Regular practice helps to increase joint flexibility, reduce stiffness, and alleviate pain associated with conditions like arthritis. The gentle stretching and strengthening exercises improve muscle tone and stability, reducing the risk of falls and injuries. Additionally, chair yoga promotes cardiovascular health by encouraging deep, mindful breathing and moderate aerobic activity, helping to maintain a healthy heart and circulatory system.

Beyond the physical benefits, chair yoga offers significant mental and emotional advantages. The practice incorporates mindfulness and meditation techniques that help reduce stress, anxiety, and depression. For men navigating the often challenging transitions of midlife, chair yoga provides a sanctuary of calm and introspection. The focus on breath control and mental clarity enhances cognitive function, helping to maintain sharpness and improve memory. This holistic approach to health ensures that you not only stay fit but also cultivate a peaceful and resilient mind.

One of the most appealing aspects of chair yoga is its versatility and adaptability. It can be practiced virtually anywhere, whether at home, in the office, or at a community center, making it a convenient addition to any lifestyle. The exercises can be easily modified to suit individual needs and fitness levels, ensuring that everyone can participate and benefit, regardless of their physical condition. This inclusivity makes chair yoga a sustainable and enjoyable practice that can be continued well into the later years of life.

Chair yoga not only improves health but also creates a sense of belonging and community. Engaging in a chair yoga class or group can offer beneficial social interaction—especially for senior citizens who might otherwise feel alone. Sharing the experience with others creates a supportive environment where individuals can connect, share experiences, and encourage each other on their wellness journeys.

Embracing chair yoga is not just about maintaining health; it's about enhancing the quality of life. The combination of physical exercise, mental clarity, and emotional balance creates a foundation for a vibrant and fulfilling life. By dedicating time to this practice, you invest in your future self, ensuring that you remain active, independent, and full of vitality as you age.

www.ingramcontent.com/pod-product-compliance
Lightning Source LLC
Chambersburg PA
CBHW061256250726
48653CB00002B/670